MINDFULNESS MEDITATION TECHNIQUES

A Comprehensive Guide To Breath Awareness, Body Scan, Walking Meditation, Loving-Kindness Meditation, And Mindful Eating For Enhanced Well-Being And Self-Discovery

WILFREDO CARSON

INTRODUCTION 3

CHAPTER 1 ....**10**

FOUNDATIONS OF MINDFULNESS........10

CHAPTER 2 ....**15**

GETTING STARTED..............................15

CHAPTER 3 ....**21**

ADVANCED MINDFULNESS PRACTICES..21

CHAPTER 4 ....**27**

OVERCOMING CHALLENGES 27

CHAPTER 5 ....**34**

MINDFULNESS AND EMOTIONAL WELL-BEING 34

CHAPTER 6 ....**39**

MINDFULNESS IN EVERYDAY LIFE.........39

CHAPTER 7 ....**46**

INTEGRATING MINDFULNESS INTO YOUR LIFESTYLE...46

CONCLUSION.......................................50

INTRODUCTION

Understanding Mindful Meditation

Mindfulness meditation is a contemplative practice with significant origins in many religious and philosophical traditions. At its core, it is cultivating heightened awareness and nonjudgmental attention to the present moment. This practice enables people to examine their thoughts and feelings without attachment, which promotes a non-reactive and receptive attitude. Mindfulness meditation originated in ancient Eastern religions, particularly Buddhism.

For centuries, Buddhist teachings have emphasized the concept of mindfulness, known as "sati" in Pali and "smṛti" in Sanskrit.

Mindfulness meditation seeks to bring about a significant shift in one's connection with ideas and emotions, rather than simply relaxing the mind. Mindfulness can help people separate from automatic emotions, lessen suffering caused by mental states, and create a sense of inner calm. Mindfulness meditation has numerous benefits, which have been intensively researched in recent years.

These benefits include increased mental health, cognitive capacities, stress reduction, and greater emotional management. The practice has acquired popularity outside of its original religious and cultural contexts, with applicability in a variety of secular settings and therapeutic procedures.

Mindfulness meditation has profound origins in contemplative traditions, and its intellectual underpinnings are based on Eastern philosophy. The practice's incorporation into Buddhist teachings can be traced back to Siddhartha Gautama, the Buddha, who emphasized mindfulness as a means to enlightenment. Throughout the years, many Buddhist schools have developed diverse meditation techniques, each emphasizing the development of attentive awareness. These practices were traditionally passed down orally and experientially from teacher to student, adding to the diverse range of mindfulness meditation techniques available today.

<u>Importance in Modern Life.</u>

Mindfulness meditation has gained popularity in recent years due to its importance in managing the challenges of a fast-paced, technologically driven environment.

As society grows more networked and the pace of life quickens, individuals are frequently overwhelmed by stress, worry, and an endless flood of information. Mindfulness meditation is a practical and accessible tool for people to handle these obstacles by increasing present-moment awareness and mental resilience.

Mindfulness in a Fast-paced World

The modern world's hectic pace, marked by continual connectedness and information overload, has sparked a renewed interest in mindfulness meditation as a means of achieving balance and peace. Work pressures, social obligations, and digital distractions are frequently associated with increased stress and decreased well-being.

Mindfulness offers a counterbalance by urging people to slow down, pay attention to their thoughts and emotions, and live in the present now. This conscious awareness enables a more effective response to stressors and obstacles, producing a sense of peace and clarity amidst the chaos of modern life.

Scientific Backing

The growing popularity of mindfulness meditation in mainstream culture has inspired substantial scientific research into its effectiveness and impact on mental health. Numerous research have shown that mindfulness meditation improves many areas of well-being. Neuroscientific research, in particular, has revealed insights into the neural systems that underpin mindfulness practices. Functional magnetic resonance imaging (fMRI) studies have indicated that regular mindfulness meditation can cause structural changes in the brain, notably in areas related to attention, emotional control, and self-awareness.

Mindfulness meditation has been scientifically validated, which has helped it integrate into conventional treatment practices. Mindfulness-Based Stress Reduction (MBSR) and Mindfulness-Based Cognitive Therapy (MBCT) are evidence-based programs that use mindfulness concepts to treat disorders like anxiety, depression, and chronic pain. These structured programs have been widely adopted in clinical settings, demonstrating mindfulness's transformative potential for improving mental health and well-being.

Mindfulness meditation is a profound and ancient technique that is extremely relevant in the present world. Its roots in Eastern traditions, along with a growing body of scientific evidence confirming its advantages, make it an adaptable tool for improving mental health and managing the obstacles of modern life. As people look for effective stress management and well-being solutions, mindfulness meditation stands out as a time-tested and scientifically verified method for developing a deeper connection with the present moment and a more resilient mind.

CHAPTER 1
FOUNDATIONS OF MINDFULNESS

Mindfulness philosophy provides the foundation for understanding and implementing mindfulness meditation practices.

Mindfulness is based on ancient contemplative traditions, particularly Buddhism, and has received considerable acceptance in modern psychology and health practices. The philosophy focuses on building a higher level of awareness and presence in the present moment. Mindfulness is the deliberate and nonjudgmental attention to one's thoughts, feelings, and experiences. The Four Foundations of Mindfulness, as defined in Buddhist teachings, offer an organized framework for mindfulness practice.

These foundations include mindfulness of the body, feelings, mind, and phenomena. Each foundation provides a pathway to greater self-awareness, promoting a comprehensive comprehension of one's inner experiences.

Cultivating awareness is an important part of mindfulness philosophy.

This entails cultivating great sensitivity to the present moment, which enables people to notice their thoughts and feelings without reacting. Awareness goes beyond the surface level, helping people to explore the complexities of their inner world. Mindfulness teaches the art of being present in the now without getting caught up in the past or thinking ahead.

Cultivating awareness entails developing an open and accepting mindset, which serves as the foundation for a transformative journey toward greater self-knowledge and emotional regulation.

Mindfulness versus Meditation

The line between mindfulness and meditation is frequently blurred, leading to uncertainty concerning their exact meanings and applications. Clarifying terminology is critical for a comprehensive understanding of these issues. Mindfulness, in essence, refers to the attribute of being fully present and engaged in the moment. It is a mental condition defined by increased awareness and nonjudgmental observation. Meditation, on the other hand, is a broader phrase that refers to a variety of techniques and practices used to achieve mental clarity, relaxation, or heightened consciousness.

Mindfulness meditation, then, can be defined as a type of meditation that focuses on developing mindfulness.

The relationship and distinctions between mindfulness and meditation add to a thorough understanding of these practices.

While mindfulness can be developed through a variety of daily activities, meditation provides a concentrated time and space for structured practice. Meditation offers a controlled environment in which people can improve their mindfulness skills, frequently using specific techniques like focused attention, loving-kindness, or body scan meditations.

Understanding the symbiotic relationship between mindfulness and meditation allows practitioners to smoothly incorporate these practices into their daily lives, cultivating a harmonious balance of heightened awareness in both formal and informal situations.

CHAPTER 2
GETTING STARTED

<u>Setting the Stage.</u>

Setting the atmosphere for mindfulness meditation entails creating an environment that supports focused and intentional practice. This goes beyond simply finding a peaceful spot; it includes the concept of creating a hallowed space. In the context of mindfulness, a sacred space is a specified area that serves as a sanctuary for one's practice. This area is purposely free of distractions and disruptions, generating a sense of calm and focus. It could be a room, a section of a room, or even an outdoor location that speaks to the practitioner. This concept is based on ancient traditions, which held that creating a sacred place was necessary for interacting with the spiritual realm. In the modern context, it serves as a physical manifestation of the commitment to mindfulness, alerting the mind that it is time to enter a state of presence.

In addition to creating a sacred environment, rituals play an important role in preparing for mindfulness meditation. Rituals give purpose to the practice by marking the start and end of each session. These rituals can take many forms, such as lighting a candle, burning incense, or simply pausing to express appreciation. The repetition of rituals signals to the mind that it is entering a new level of consciousness. Over time, these rituals become brain cues, making it easier to transition into mindfulness practice. By including rituals, people can build an organized and intentional framework for their meditation sessions, improving the entire experience and increasing their commitment to the practice.

<u>Basic Mindfulness Techniques</u>

Basic mindfulness practices form the cornerstone of meditation practice, helping people to build essential abilities for cultivating present-moment awareness. Among these strategies, breath awareness stands out as a foundational practice.

Breath awareness entails drawing one's attention to the natural rhythm of the breath.

This approach is based on the notion that the breath acts as a grounding force in the present moment, helping people to center themselves and examine their thoughts without becoming caught in them. By focusing on the breath, practitioners develop a more acute sense of awareness, learning to watch the ebb and flow of their thoughts and emotions without judgment.

Another fundamental approach is the body scan, which entails carefully directing attention to various regions of the body.

The body scan is a type of mindfulness practice that promotes a nonjudgmental awareness of bodily sensations, resulting in a strong connection between the mind and body.

This technique is very useful for those looking to relieve tension and stress accumulated in various regions of the body. As people proceed through the body scan, they become more sensitive to the subtle subtleties of physical experiences, leading to a better awareness of the mind-body link.

Loving-kindness meditation, also known as "Metta" meditation, is another important mindfulness method that focuses on developing compassion and love for oneself and others. This practice entails repeating statements or affirmations that convey benevolence and positive purpose. Practitioners cultivate a compassionate and empathy-filled mindset by first aiming for loving-kindness towards themselves and then expanding it to others. This strategy not only improves emotional well-being but also promotes the formation of positive interpersonal relationships. Loving-kindness meditation is an effective strategy for overcoming boundaries and fostering a sense of connectivity with all living beings.

To summarize, fundamental mindfulness techniques give a great basis for anybody starting on a meditation journey. These practices, which include breath awareness, body scan, and loving-kindness meditation, provide a variety of approaches to building mindfulness, allowing practitioners to select techniques that best suit their tastes and goals. Individuals who engage in these core practices regularly can lay the groundwork for more advanced and specialized kinds of mindfulness meditation.

CHAPTER 3
ADVANCED MINDFULNESS PRACTICES

1. Walking Meditation

Walking meditation is a unique and advanced mindfulness technique in which you cultivate awareness while walking. Individuals who use this approach pay close attention to each step, developing a strong connection between the mind and body. One important feature is "Mindful Movement," in which practitioners synchronize their breath with each stride, resulting in a greater awareness of the present moment. This synchronization not only improves focus but also helps to ground oneself in the present experience. Furthermore, practitioners investigate the nuances of movement, such as weight shifting and the sensation of feet touching the ground.

Walking meditation's emphasis on attentive movement bridges the gap between traditional seated meditation and daily activities, providing a unique viewpoint on how to integrate mindfulness into one's life.

Furthermore, "Integrating Awareness into Daily Activities" is an important part of walking meditation. This approach is based on expanding the principles of mindfulness beyond regular practice sessions. Practitioners learn to incorporate mindfulness into everyday activities, such as walking to work, standing in line, and performing ordinary tasks.

This integration enhances mindfulness's transformative power by weaving it into the fabric of daily living. By incorporating mindfulness into everyday activities, people not only increase their overall awareness but also create a profound sense of presence in each moment. The walking meditation technique, which focuses on both movement and daily integration, is an advanced practice that promotes a comprehensive approach to mindfulness.

2. Mindful Eating

Mindful eating is a nuanced activity that extends beyond simply eating food. It explores the complex relationship between the mind, body, and food, emphasizing a conscious and purposeful approach to eating. "Savoring the Present Moment" is a key component of mindful eating, encouraging people to use all of their senses in the meal experience.

This entails appreciating the colors, textures, and scents of the meal, and developing a strong connection to the process of eating. Practitioners purposefully slow down their eating pace, allowing them to relish each bite and thoroughly appreciate the sustenance offered by the food.

In addition to sensory appreciation, mindful eating entails comprehending the psychological components of hunger and satiation. This includes identifying emotional triggers for eating and distinguishing between actual bodily hunger and other urges.

By increasing this awareness, people can make more mindful decisions about when, what, and how much to consume, resulting in a healthier relationship with food. "Developing Healthy Eating Habits" is a related topic that examines the broader impact of mindfulness on food decisions. Mindful eating promotes a nonjudgmental awareness of food choices, resulting in a more balanced and intuitive approach to nutrition. This goes beyond restrictive diets and emphasizes listening to the body's natural signals, which promotes long-term and healthy eating habits. Mindful eating, as a comprehensive practice, benefits both physical and mental health.

Advanced mindfulness techniques, such as walking meditation and mindful dining, provide important insights into incorporating awareness throughout daily life. These approaches go beyond typical sitting meditation, giving practitioners skills to increase mindfulness while moving and eating. The ideas of mindful movement and integration into daily activities in walking meditation, as well as relishing the present moment and creating good eating habits in mindful eating, all contribute to a holistic understanding of mindfulness.

These advanced practices encourage people to adopt mindfulness as a way of life, promoting overall well-being and a stronger connection to the present moment.

CHAPTER 4
OVERCOMING CHALLENGES

Dealing with Distractions: Mindfulness meditation frequently faces hurdles in the form of distractions, which can interrupt the practitioner's focus and limit the depth of their meditation experience. Common obstacles include wandering thoughts, external stimuli, and physical discomfort. The wandering mind is a common problem, as thoughts and concerns from daily life can disrupt the meditative state.

External noises, whether from the outside world or from within, might break the tranquility essential for effective meditation. Furthermore, physical discomfort, such as restlessness or pain in various body areas, might draw attention away from the present moment.

These difficulties are not uncommon, and identifying them is critical for establishing successful solutions to address them.

Common Challenges in Meditation: One of the primary challenges in meditation is the constant stream of thoughts that bombard the mind, also known as the "monkey mind."

This phenomenon involves the mind jumping from one thought to the next, making it difficult for individuals to maintain sustained focus. Another problem is the desire to resist or condemn thoughts and feelings that occur during meditation.

This resistance can be frustrating and slow down overall mindfulness progress. Furthermore, many practitioners struggle with the physical obstacle of sitting for an extended amount of time.

Understanding these common difficulties is critical for developing personalized strategies to address them systematically.

attention tactics: Several tactics can be used to reduce distractions and improve attention while practicing mindfulness meditation.

One helpful way is to acknowledge distracting ideas without judgment and gently redirect the focus back to the breath or the chosen subject of attention. This approach promotes non-reactive awareness, enabling thoughts to pass without becoming caught in them.

Another option is to incorporate mindfulness techniques into everyday tasks, eventually expanding the practice beyond formal meditation sessions.

Individuals who practice mindfulness in numerous aspects of their lives can improve their capacity to focus during devoted meditation periods.

Additionally, setting a dedicated and comfortable meditation area, reducing external disturbances, and doing deep-breathing exercises can all help to increase attention and make meditation more enjoyable.

<u>Patience and persistence:</u>

Accepting Imperfection: Patience and perseverance are essential components of an effective mindfulness meditation practice. Accepting imperfection is an essential component of developing patience in meditation.

Many people may become disappointed or discouraged when they are unable to maintain perfect attention or see instant results. Understanding that imperfection is a natural aspect of the meditation journey encourages practitioners to approach their practice with more compassion and patience. Accepting that the mind may wander and that challenges will come allows people to manage the learning curve with grit.

Building Consistent Practice: Consistency is essential for receiving the long-term benefits of mindfulness meditation. Developing a consistent and sustained meditation program involves deliberate work and dedication. Setting realistic goals and expectations is an important step in developing consistency. Beginning with modest lengths and progressively increasing meditation time can help people avoid burnout and dissatisfaction. Creating a regular timetable that incorporates meditation into daily life promotes a feeling of rhythm and increases the practice's sustainability. Furthermore, experimenting with different meditation techniques and finding one that suits personal preferences increases the likelihood of keeping a consistent practice. Understanding the cyclical nature of progress, where shifts in emphasis and experiences are normal, emphasizes the significance of perseverance in the face of adversity.

Mindfulness meditation is a transforming technique that necessitates a deliberate approach to overcome obstacles and acquire vital qualities like focus, patience, and perseverance. Practitioners can deepen their meditation experience by recognizing common problems, such as distractions, and employing effective methods.

Accepting imperfection and maintaining a consistent practice are critical components of developing patience and tenacity, which ensures mindfulness meditation's long-term effectiveness as a valuable tool for personal growth and well-being.

CHAPTER 5
MINDFULNESS AND EMOTIONAL WELL-BEING

Mindfulness meditation improves emotional well-being by building emotional intelligence. This entails gaining a better understanding of one's own emotions and the capacity to navigate them effectively. Individuals seeking emotional intelligence participate in mindfulness activities that promote emotional recognition and acceptance. This technique entails acknowledging and comprehending emotions without passing judgment, resulting in a more balanced and compassionate relationship with oneself. Mindfulness-based emotional intelligence development improves emotional regulation and increases empathy for others.

Furthermore, in the field of emotional intelligence, the concept of responding vs reacting is an essential component of mindfulness meditation. Responding requires taking a thoughtful and intentional attitude to emotional stimuli, allowing people to make conscious decisions about their behaviors.

In contrast, reacting is frequently impulsive and automatic, motivated by instinctive emotional responses. Mindfulness meditation encourages people to examine their emotions rather than react to them right away. This increased self-awareness allows for more intentional reactions, resulting in better interpersonal connections and overall emotional well-being.

Stress Reduction:

Mindfulness meditation is generally acknowledged for its stress-reduction benefits, providing a holistic approach to dealing with the complexities of stressors in everyday life. The relationship between mindfulness and the stress response is a critical component of this phenomenon. Mindfulness activities help people acquire the ability to observe their thoughts and emotions without becoming involved in them. This nonjudgmental awareness establishes a psychological distance from stressors, lowering the severity of the stress reaction and encouraging a more balanced mental state.

Mindfulness-Based Stress Reduction (MBSR) is one-way mindfulness can be used to reduce stress. Jon Kabat-Zinn created MBSR, a structured program that combines mindfulness meditation and yoga to reduce stress and improve overall well-being. Participants engage in mindfulness techniques, body scan meditations, and mild yoga to promote a comprehensive approach to stress management. Numerous studies have found that MBSR reduces perceived stress and anxiety while improving overall mental health.

To reduce stress through mindfulness, it is necessary to investigate the physiological and psychological mechanisms that underpin this transforming process. Mindfulness meditation has been linked to changes in brain structure and function, notably in areas involving stress regulation and emotional processing.

These neural modifications help to boost resilience and provide a more balanced response to stressors, emphasizing the complex interplay between mindfulness and stress neuroscience.

mindfulness meditation is an effective stress-reduction method because it promotes non-reactive awareness of thoughts and emotions. The incorporation of mindfulness practices, as demonstrated by MBSR, offers individuals practical and systematic techniques for stress management. Mindfulness stands out as a holistic stress-reduction method due to its emphasis on awareness and proactive participation, which has far-reaching implications for mental health and well-being.

CHAPTER 6
MINDFULNESS IN EVERYDAY LIFE

Mindfulness in everyday life is a comprehensive method of incorporating mindfulness practices into daily activities, developing a greater sense of awareness and presence in each moment. It moves beyond formal meditation sessions and becomes a way of life, influencing many facets of existence. This notion focuses on building mindfulness in everyday tasks, turning ordinary moments into opportunities for self-awareness and conscious living.

<u>Relationship and Communication:</u>

In terms of relationships and communication, mindfulness is critical for building deeper connections and understanding.

 Mindful listening, a key component of good communication, is completely immersing oneself in the current moment during interactions. This exercise encourages empathy, patience, and true connections with others. Another aspect of compassionate communication is expressing oneself with empathy and understanding, which promotes a healthy exchange of thoughts and feelings. It turns disagreements into opportunities for mutual progress, highlighting the significance of awareness in interpersonal dynamics.

Mindful Listening:

Mindful listening is a skill that entails being fully present and engaged with the speaker.

This practice involves cultivating an open, nonjudgmental awareness of the speaker's words, tone, and body language. Mindful listening, which suspends preconceived assumptions and internal chatter, enables for a more in-depth grasp of the speaker's perspective. It fosters trust and deepens relationships by demonstrating genuine interest in the other person's experiences and feelings. Mindful listening improves communication by promoting sincerity and mutual regard.

<u>Compassionate Communication:</u>

Compassionate communication, based on awareness, changes the way people express themselves and respond to others. It entails expressing thoughts and feelings with clarity and empathy while creating a happy and supportive environment.

This method enables people to communicate from a position of understanding rather than a response. Compassionate communication reduces conflict and encourages collaborative problem-solving by acknowledging and affirming feelings. It improves relationships by fostering an environment of empathy in which everyone feels heard and appreciated.

<u>Work and productivity:</u>

Mindfulness in the context of work and productivity means bringing conscious awareness to professional duties, optimizing focus, and improving general well-being at work. It goes beyond the typical idea of work as only a means to an end, emphasizing the significance of being fully present and involved in the workplace.

<u>Mindfulness in the workplace:</u>

Mindfulness in the workplace entails incorporating mindfulness practices to foster a work culture that values both well-being and productivity. This notion acknowledges the link between employee mental health and company success. Mindful firms create a supportive environment in which employees are encouraged to devote their entire attention to tasks, resulting in higher job satisfaction and lower stress. Mindfulness at work includes activities such as attentive breathing, taking short meditation breaks, and developing a nonjudgmental awareness of one's tasks. This technique not only improves individual performance but also promotes a positive organizational culture.

Improving focus and creativity:

Mindfulness is an effective strategy for increasing focus and creativity in the business world. Individuals can overcome distractions by training their minds to be fully present, resulting in increased attention. Mindfulness promotes creativity by cultivating an open, inquiring, and receptive mindset to new ideas. This element entails implementing mindfulness practices into daily work routines, such as mindful breaks, mindful walks, or short meditation sessions. As a result, employees are encouraged to innovate, solve problems, and have a sense of purpose at work.

Mindfulness in daily life has a wide range of applications, influencing how people interact with themselves, others, and their work.

The notions of attentive listening, compassionate communication, mindfulness in the workplace, and improving focus and creativity are all interrelated threads in a tapestry of conscious living. Individuals and organizations that practice mindfulness in these dimensions can build a harmonic balance between productivity and well-being, promoting a culture of awareness, compassion, and long-term success.

CHAPTER 7
INTEGRATING MINDFULNESS INTO YOUR LIFESTYLE

Mindfulness meditation has grown in popularity due to its ability to improve general well-being and lead to a more fulfilling existence. Individuals who begin the road of incorporating mindfulness into their lives gain access to a plethora of long-term advantages. One of the most important characteristics of mindfulness is its potential to encourage a holistic approach to health, encompassing both physical and mental well-being. This section examines the profound and long-term benefits of mindfulness meditation.

Long-term Benefits:

Mindfulness and Physical Health: Mindfulness meditation has been connected to multiple physical health advantages, proving its influence on various areas of the human body. According to studies, regular mindfulness meditation can help with cardiovascular health by lowering blood pressure and improving heart function. Furthermore, mindfulness has been linked to a stronger immune system, which improves the body's ability to defend against infections. The practice's stress-reduction effects are critical in promoting general physical health, as chronic stress has been linked to a variety of health problems, including inflammation and a weakened immune system.

Mental Well-Being and Resilience: Studies have consistently shown that mindfulness meditation improves mental health.

Mindfulness techniques have been demonstrated to reduce symptoms of anxiety and despair, giving people a tool to manage and minimize these frequent mental health difficulties. Furthermore, mindfulness promotes emotional resilience, allowing people to handle life's ups and downs with greater calm. Mindfulness practice has been linked to changes in brain structure and function, notably in areas such as attention, emotion management, and self-awareness, all of which contribute to improved mental well-being over time.

<u>Setting Up a Mindfulness Practice:</u>

Tailoring Practices to Your Preferences: Personalizing practices is an important part of successful mindfulness integration. Mindfulness is not a one-size-fits-all strategy, and understanding this helps people to select practices that speak to them uniquely.

Whether it's mindfulness meditation, mindful breathing exercises, or mindful movement practices like yoga, personalizing the routine to individual tastes increases the likelihood of long-term participation. This adaptability ensures that mindfulness becomes a natural and joyful part of one's daily routine, boosting the possibility of long-term commitment and reaping the benefits.

Overcoming Resistance: Despite the potential benefits, people frequently experience resistance while attempting to create a mindfulness program. Overcoming this resistance is critical to properly incorporating mindfulness into one's daily life. One typical barrier is the assumption that mindfulness necessitates a considerable time investment.

In actuality, even short daily routines can provide significant benefits. Additionally, addressing myths and demystifying mindfulness might help minimize resistance. Educating people about the flexibility of mindfulness practices and debunking myths can help to create a more inclusive and accessible environment in which people can incorporate mindfulness into their daily lives.

CONCLUSION

Mindfulness meditation practices provide a comprehensive approach to improving total well-being by addressing physical health, mental health, and resilience. The long-term advantages of mindfulness go beyond the individual, potentially influencing social well-being by cultivating healthier individuals who are better able to face life's problems. Integrating mindfulness into one's lifestyle necessitates a personalized approach that tailors' practices to individual preferences while also overcoming opposition through education and myth-busting. Individuals who engage on this journey are opening themselves up to the profound and long-term benefits of mindfulness, creating a life of physical health, mental well-being, and emotional resilience.

www.ingramcontent.com/pod-product-compliance
Lightning Source LLC
Chambersburg PA
CBHW060813260726

48660CB00002B/922